A WARRIOR'S JOURNEY

A Guided Journal To Reflect On Your Well-Being

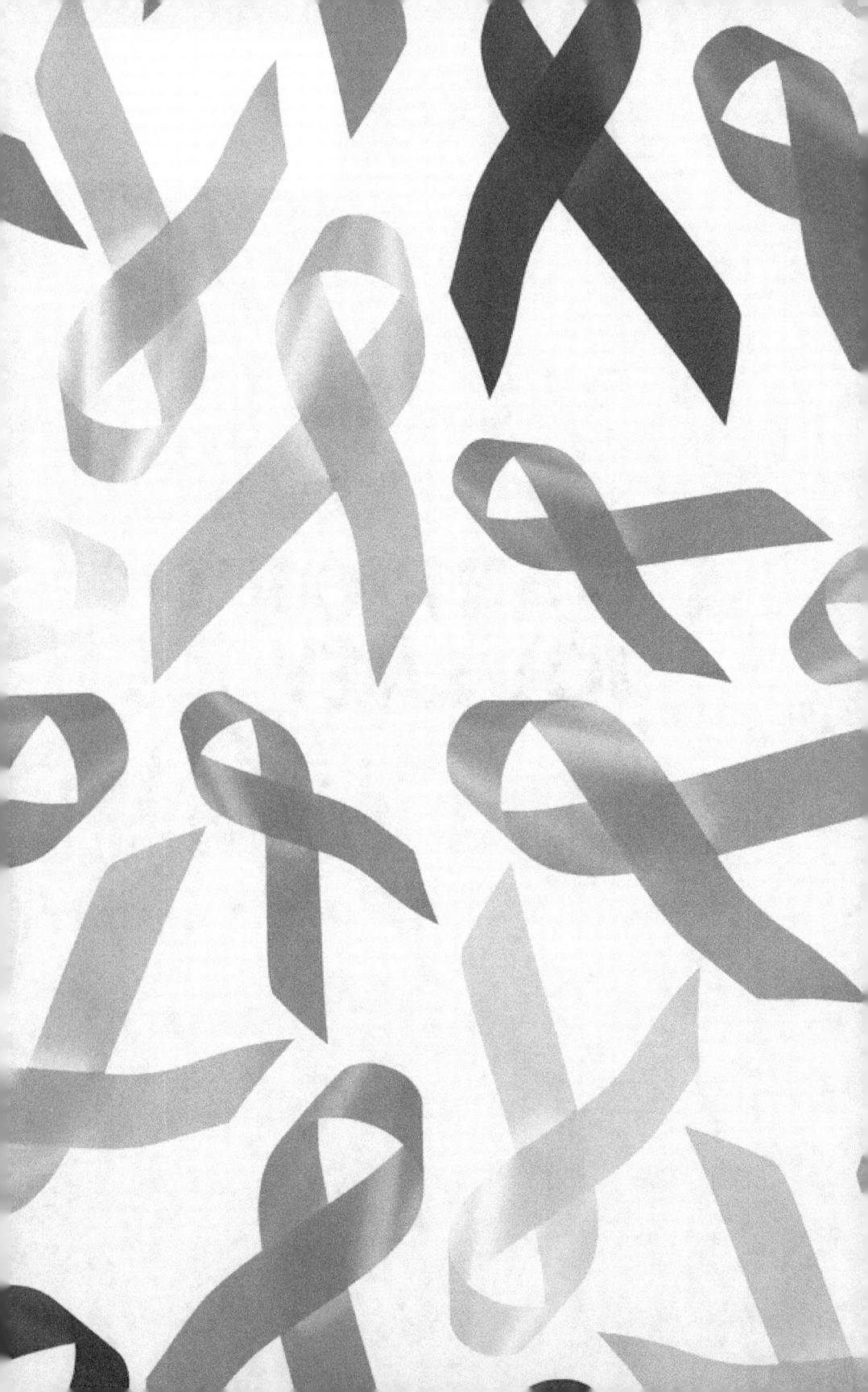

I dedicate this book to all cancer warriors. You are strong and a fighter!

ISBN: 978-1-7367038-5-4

Copyright © 2021 by Flor Publishing LLC
Written by Marci Greenberg Cox
All Rights Reserved
www.florpublishing.com

No part of this book may be used or reproduced in any manner whatsoever without the prior written permission of the author.

Introduction

I created this journal to really make you think about your life, your journey, and your diagnosis.

What have you done differently with your life now that you have received a cancer diagnosis?

Each page throughout the journal has questions to help you organize your thoughts and ideas. You can write your thoughts down or choose from a list of words to help express your feelings.

When you're ready, come back and read your writing and reflect on any growth you have experienced or any areas which still need attention. Ask yourself questions like, "Have I implemented the changes into my life which I thought were important? What areas do I still need to work on or focus more attention toward?"

-Marci Greenberg Cox

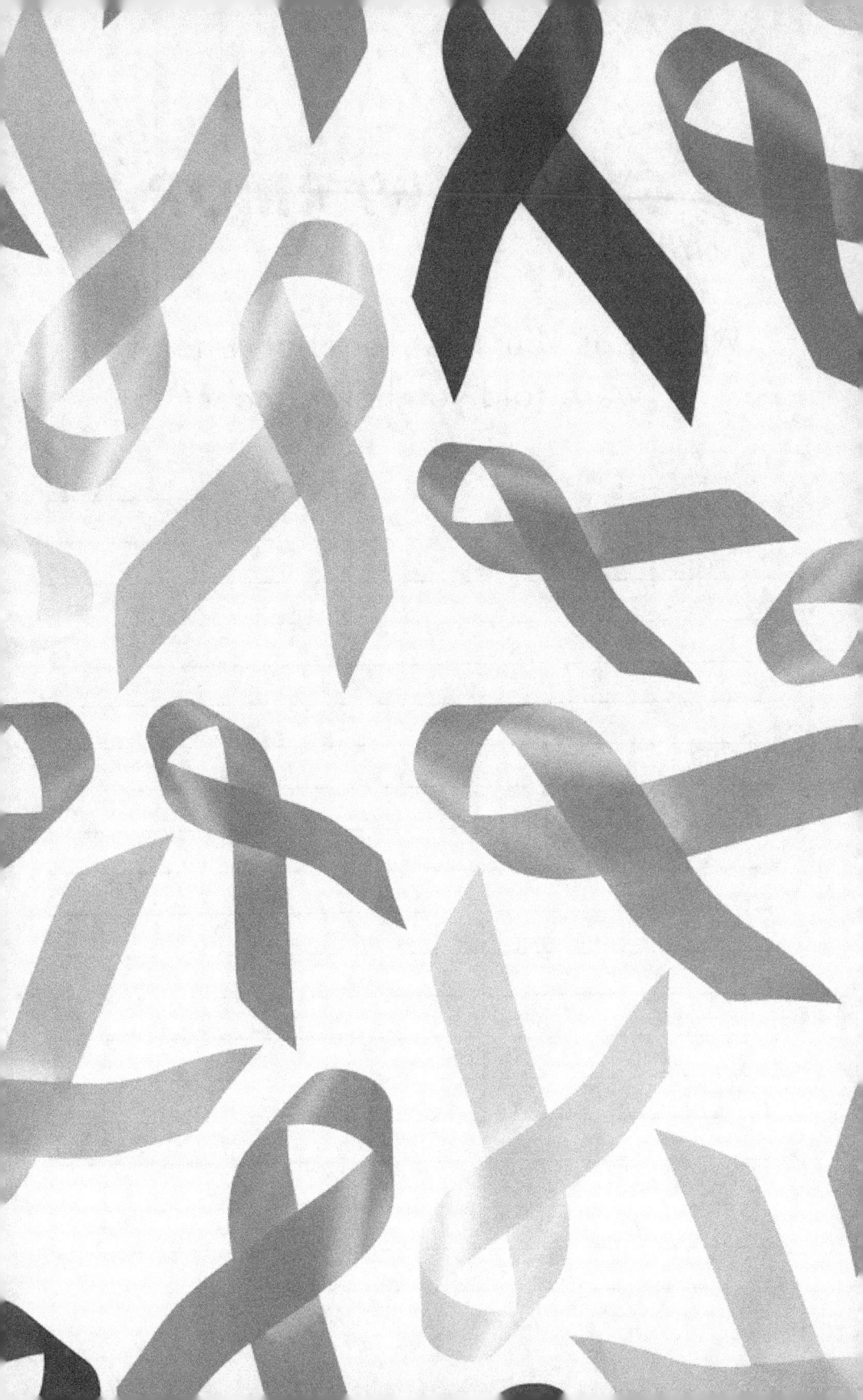

CANCER WARRIOR

What was your first reaction when you were told you had cancer?

Date:_____

Date:_____

_____
_____
_____
_____
_____
_____
_____
_____
_____
_____
_____
_____
_____
_____
_____
_____
_____
_____
_____
_____
_____
_____
_____
_____
_____
_____
_____

SHOCKED   TERRIFIED CONFUSED   ANGRY

SCARED   SAD WORRIED MAD SELF-ACCEPTING

STRONG RESILIENT CALM LIFELESS   PEACEFUL

CANCER WARRIOR

Is there family history of cancer? Who in your family has had cancer?

Date:_____

Date:_____

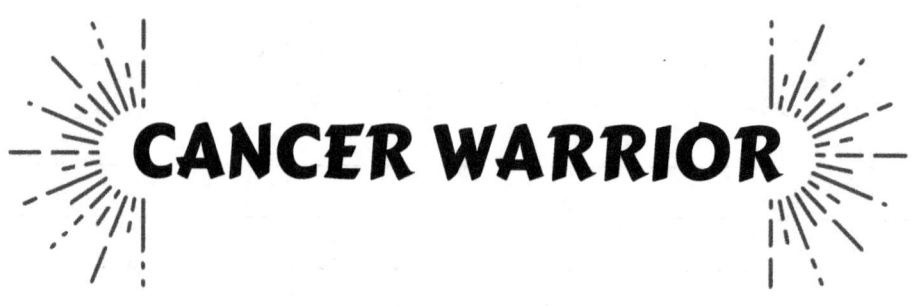

CANCER WARRIOR

Did you/have you joined a support group? If so, has it helped?

Date:_____

Date:_____

ANXIOUS SAD WORRIED TOUGH CONFUSED
SCARED UNDERSTANDING ANGRY SELF-ACCEPTING
STRONG CALM PEACEFUL TERRIFIED QUIET

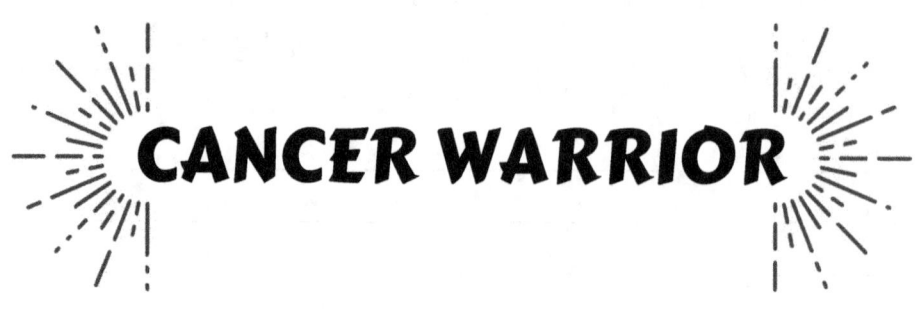

CANCER WARRIOR

Have you changed anything with your physical or mental health?

Date:_____

Date:_____

_____
_____
_____
_____
_____
_____
_____
_____
_____
_____
_____
_____
_____
_____
_____
_____
_____
_____
_____
_____
_____
_____
_____
_____
_____
_____

SHOCKED   HAPPY   SCARED   WORRIED   STRONG
CRABBY   CONFUSED   ANNOYED   TERRIFIED   EASY
TOUGH   SELF-ACCEPTING   PEACEFUL   CALM

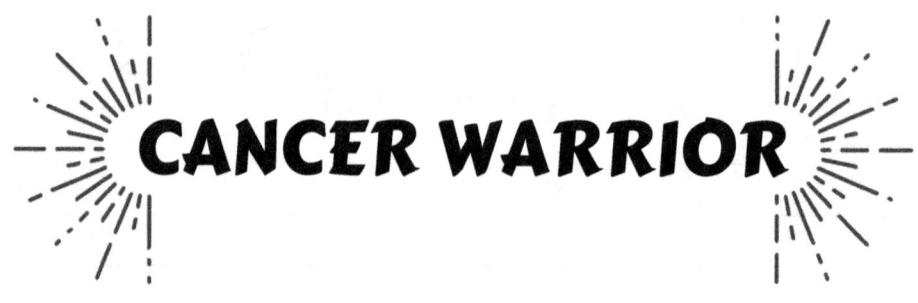

CANCER WARRIOR

How did you approach your treatments?

Date:_____

Date:_____

_____
_____
_____
_____
_____
_____
_____
_____
_____
_____
_____
_____
_____
_____
_____
_____
_____
_____
_____
_____
_____
_____
_____
_____
_____

HEADSTRONG   SADNESS   PEACEFUL   ANGRY

LAUGHTER   SELF-ACCEPTING   WORRIED   ALONE

CONFUSED   HOPE   SCARED   DETERMINATION

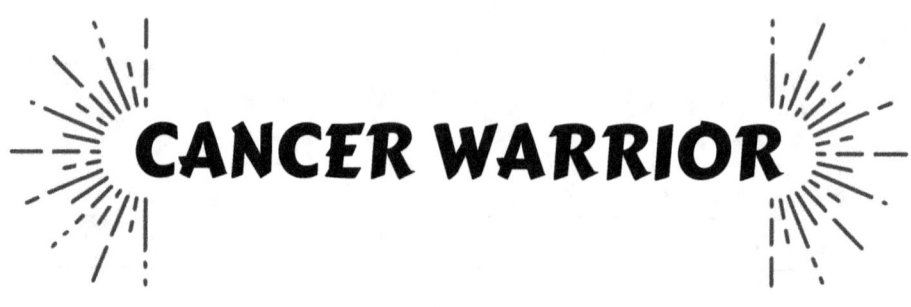

CANCER WARRIOR

What scares you about your diagnosis?

Date:_____

_____
_____
_____
_____
_____
_____
_____
_____
_____
_____
_____
_____
_____
_____
_____
_____
_____
_____
_____
_____
_____
_____

Date:_____

_____
_____
_____
_____
_____
_____
_____
_____
_____
_____
_____
_____
_____
_____
_____
_____
_____
_____
_____
_____
_____
_____
_____
_____
_____
_____

**SAD   ANGRY   SCARED   WORRIED   MAD
RESILIENT   AFRAID PANICKED CONFUSED
NERVOUS   STRONG   TERRIFIED   SHOCKED
PEACEFUL   JITTERY   TOUGH**

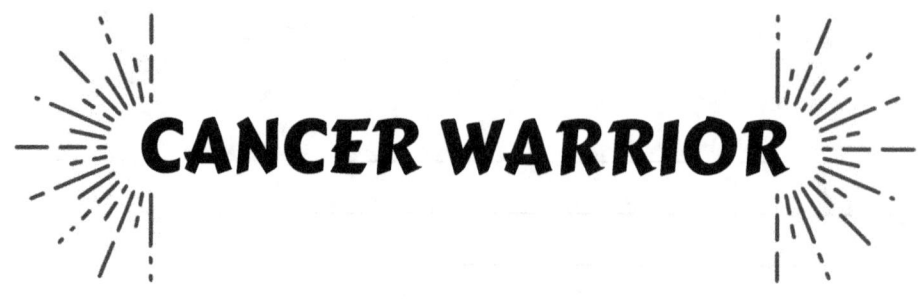

Are there any fears you have overcome since being diagnosed?

Date:_____

Date:_____

_____
_____
_____
_____
_____
_____
_____
_____
_____
_____
_____
_____
_____
_____
_____
_____
_____
_____
_____
_____
_____
_____
_____
_____

**RESILIENT COURAGE SCARED LOVE WORRIED
CONFUSED STRONG INDEPENDENT RESILIENT
CALM PEACEFUL TOUGH FAITH POSITIVE ACCEPTING**

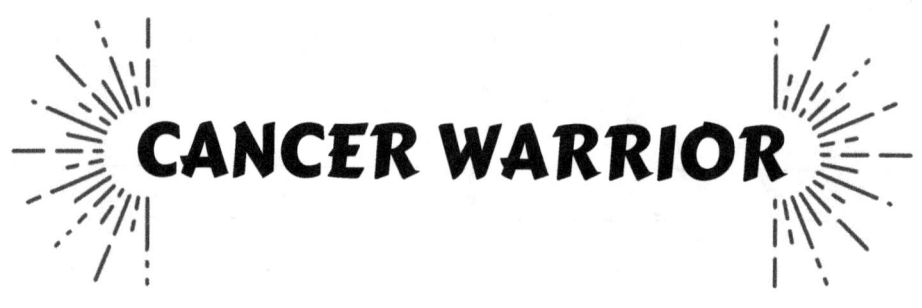

CANCER WARRIOR

Do/Did you have help from family or friends? And if, so what kind of help?

Date:_____

Date:_____

_____
_____
_____
_____
_____
_____
_____
_____
_____
_____
_____
_____
_____
_____
_____
_____
_____
_____
_____
_____
_____
_____
_____
_____

**LOVED   FRUSTRATED   DISAPPOINTED   WORRIED
SATISFIED   ALONE   STRONG   SAVED   SCARED   CALM
SUPPORTED   LET DOWN   NEEDY   TERRIFIED   ANGRY**

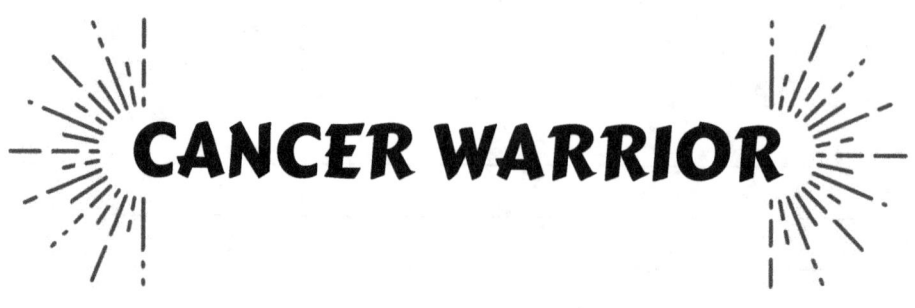

CANCER WARRIOR

What did you NOT want to hear from people?

Date:_____

Date:_____

_____

ANGRY   KIND   PEACEFUL   SELF-ACCEPTING   MAD
SCARED   WORRIED   SAD   TERRIFIED   CONFUSED
TOUGH   CALM   STRONG   RESILIENT   DISSATISFIED

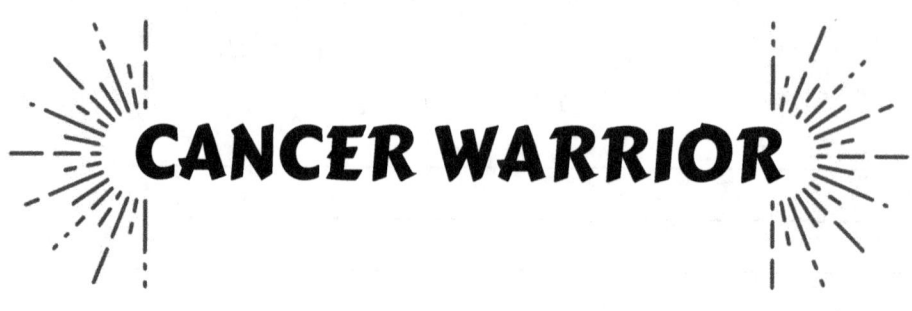

CANCER WARRIOR

What did you WANT to hear from people?

Date:_____

Date:_____

_____
_____
_____
_____
_____
_____
_____
_____
_____
_____
_____
_____
_____
_____
_____
_____
_____
_____
_____
_____
_____
_____
_____
_____

LOVED   ANGRY   SHOCKED   SAD   CONFUSED
NUTURING   WORRIED   CALM   RESILIENT   MAD
KIND   SCARED   HELPFUL   QUIET   TERRIFIED

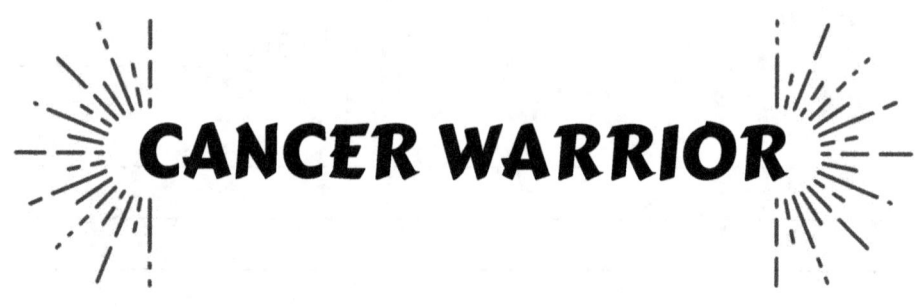

CANCER WARRIOR

Have you changed anything within you?
ie. your attitude,
how you look at things?

Date:_____

_____
_____
_____
_____
_____
_____
_____
_____
_____
_____
_____
_____
_____
_____
_____
_____
_____
_____

Date:_____

_____
_____
_____
_____
_____
_____
_____
_____
_____
_____
_____
_____
_____
_____
_____
_____
_____
_____
_____
_____
_____
_____
_____
_____
_____
_____
_____
_____

EXCITED   SCARED   MAD   SAD   WORRIED

TOUGH   OUTRAGED   LIFELESS   TERRIFIED   PLEASED

SELF-ACCEPTING   RESILIENT   FAIL   STRONG

PROSPER   CALM   TIRED   PEACEFUL

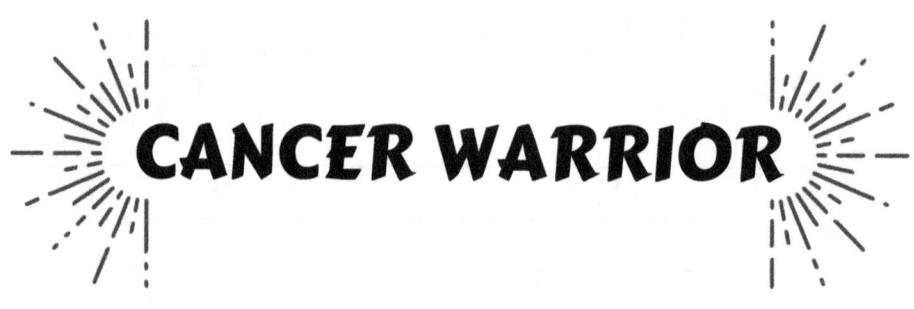

CANCER WARRIOR

What has stayed the same about you, about your life since your cancer diagnosis?

Date:_____

Date:_____

SHOCKED   SUCCEEDED   SCARED   MAD   WORRIED
SELF-ACCEPTING   STRONG   RESILIENT   PEACEFUL
CALM   TOUGH   SAD   TERRIFIED   CONFUSED   ANGRY

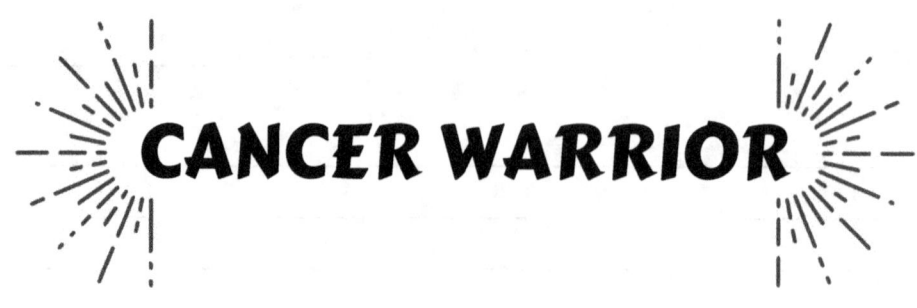

CANCER WARRIOR

In what ways has cancer made you a better person? Why?

Date:_____

Date:_____

_____
_____
_____
_____
_____
_____
_____
_____
_____
_____
_____
_____
_____
_____
_____
_____
_____
_____
_____
_____
_____
_____
_____
_____
_____

HAPPY SELF-ACCEPTING SUCCESSFUL CONFUSED
RESILIENT CALM PEACEFUL SOLID WORRIED
SCARED TOUGH DULL TERRIFIED
STRONG MAD IRRITATED

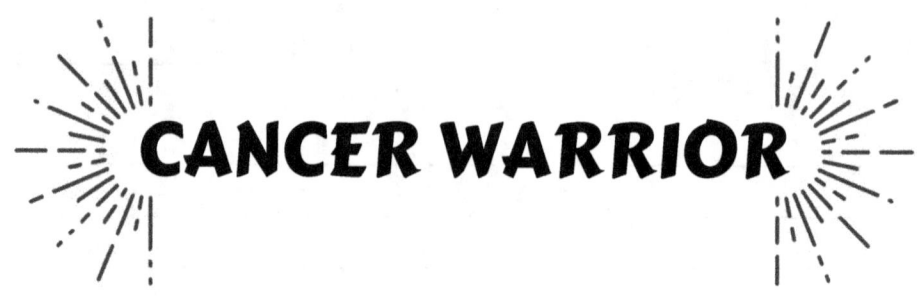

CANCER WARRIOR

Has cancer changed your life?
Why or Why not?

Date:_____

Date:_____

ANGRY   INTOXICATING   SCARED   MAD

STRONG   SELF-ACCEPTING   CALM   SHOCKED

RESILIENT   PEACEFUL   QUIET   THRILLED

CONFUSED   TERRIFIED   WORRIED

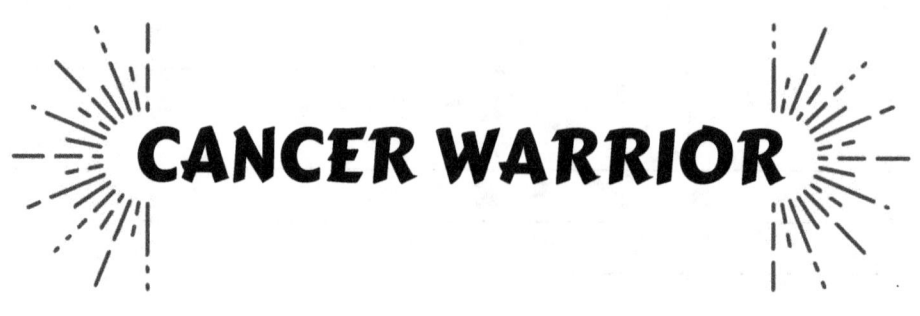

CANCER WARRIOR

Are you living life to your fullest?

Date:_____

Date:_____

_____
_____
_____
_____
_____
_____
_____
_____
_____
_____
_____
_____
_____
_____
_____
_____
_____
_____
_____
_____
_____
_____
_____
_____
_____
_____
_____
_____

SATISFIED   OVERJOYED SAD MAD   SCARED
SELF-ACCEPTING   GRATEFUL   STRONG
CALM PEACEFUL QUIET RELAXED WELL-PLEASED
TERRIFIED   CONFUSED   PRODUCTIVE

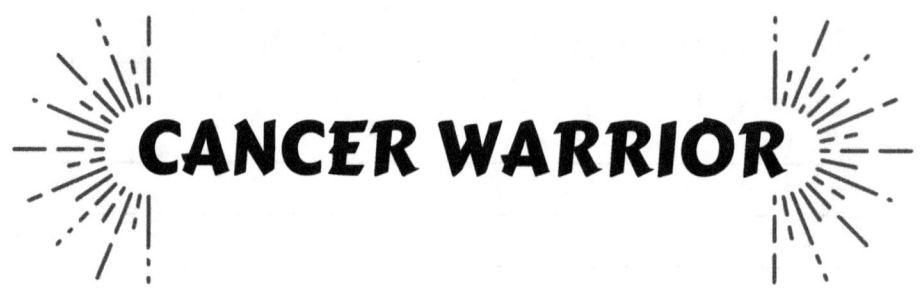

CANCER WARRIOR

How is your self-esteem?

Date:_____

_____
_____
_____
_____
_____
_____
_____
_____
_____
_____
_____
_____
_____
_____
_____
_____
_____
_____
_____
_____
_____
_____
_____
_____

Date:_____

DISPLEASED FLAT SCARED WORRIED MAD

PLEASANT SECURE CAREFREE QUIET PEACEFUL

POWERFUL CALM SELF-ACCEPTING TERRIFIED

CONFIDENT EMBARRASSED WOWED

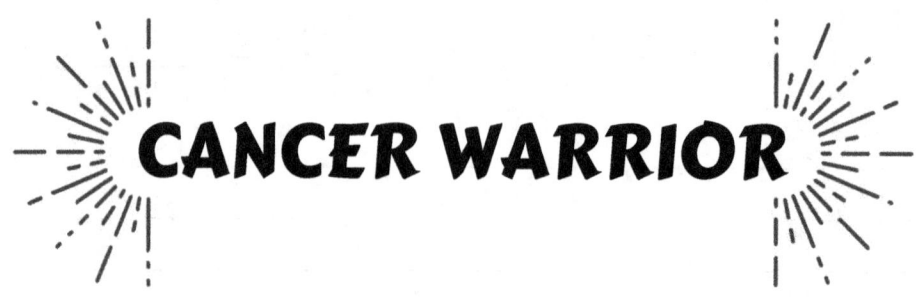

CANCER WARRIOR

Are there things which scared you before which you have now overcome?

Date:_____

Date:_____

_____
_____
_____
_____
_____
_____
_____
_____
_____
_____
_____
_____
_____
_____
_____
_____
_____
_____
_____
_____
_____
_____
_____
_____
_____
_____
_____
_____

SCARED SELF-ACCEPTING WORRIED SAD MAD
SHOCKED ANGRY CONFUSED LIFELESS CALM
TOUGH PEACEFUL QUIET TERRIFIED STRONG

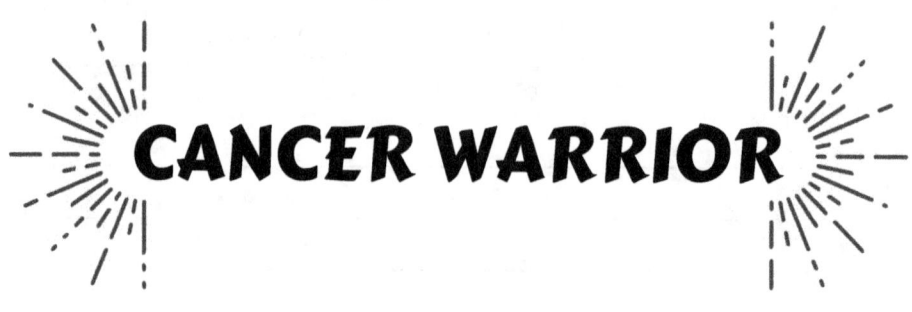

CANCER WARRIOR

What are you passionate about? If nothing, what are some things you like to do which you haven't done in a long time?

Date:_____

Date:_____

SHOCKED GIDDY ANGRY BUSY SAD STRONG
SPIRITLESS CALM LIFELESS TERRIFIED
PEACEFUL JEALOUS JOY TOUGH PLEASED
CONFUSED EXHILARATED

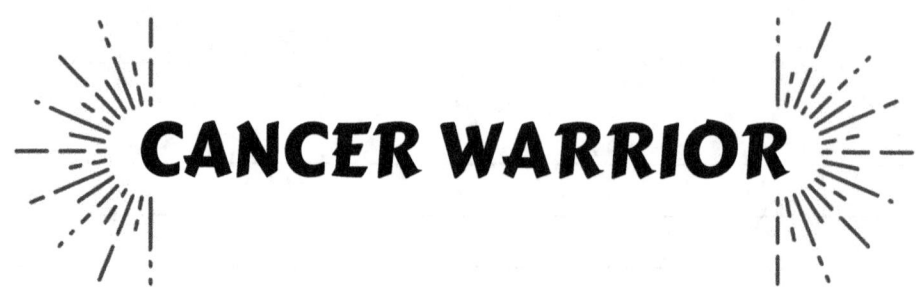

How do you define
the meaning of joy?

Date:_____

_____
_____
_____
_____
_____
_____
_____
_____
_____
_____
_____
_____
_____
_____
_____
_____
_____

Date:_____

_____
_____
_____
_____
_____
_____
_____
_____
_____
_____
_____
_____
_____
_____
_____
_____
_____
_____
_____
_____
_____
_____
_____
_____
_____
_____

SHOCKED THANKFUL ELATED HAPPY CONTENT
FLEXIBLE SOOTHING PEACEFUL HUMBLE
STRONG RESILIENT CALM CONFUSED UGLY
INTERESTED TERRIFIED LOVEABLE

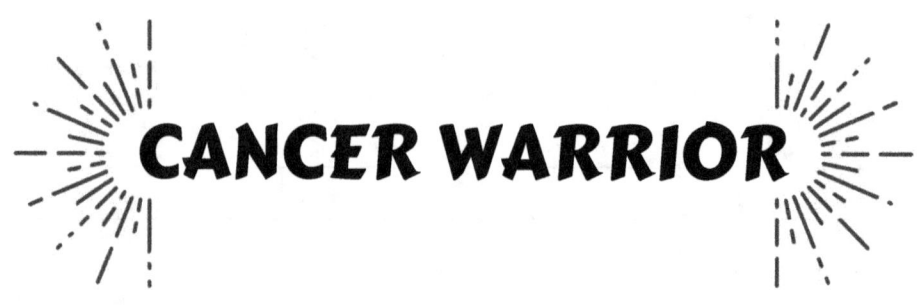

CANCER WARRIOR

How would you answer this question..
I will be happy when...?

Date:_____

Date:_____

_____
_____
_____
_____
_____
_____
_____
_____
_____
_____
_____
_____
_____
_____
_____
_____
_____
_____
_____
_____
_____
_____
_____
_____

TOUGH CALM PEACEFUL CONFIDENT DOUBTFUL
JEALOUS TERRIFIED CONFUSED SHOCKED WORRIED
ANGRY SCARED MAD SELF-ACCEPTING STRONG

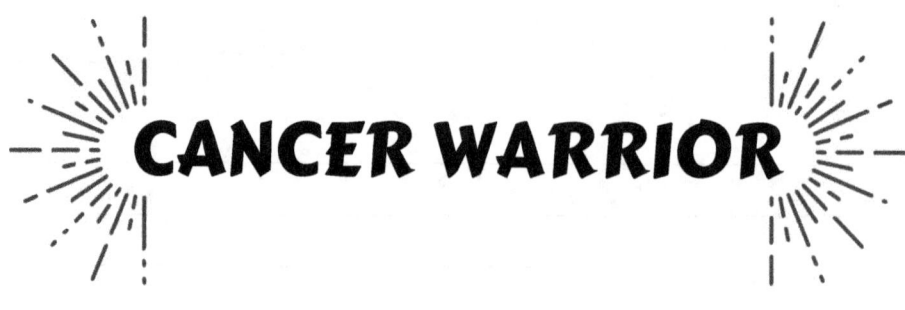

What is preventing you from being happy?

Date:_____

Date:_____

**NERVOUS SAD SCARED MAD WORRIED UNSURE
TOUGH GUILT PETRIFIED UNHAPPY CONFUSED
SELF-ACCEPTING RESILIENT PEACEFUL
STRONG CALM TERRIFIED LONELY**

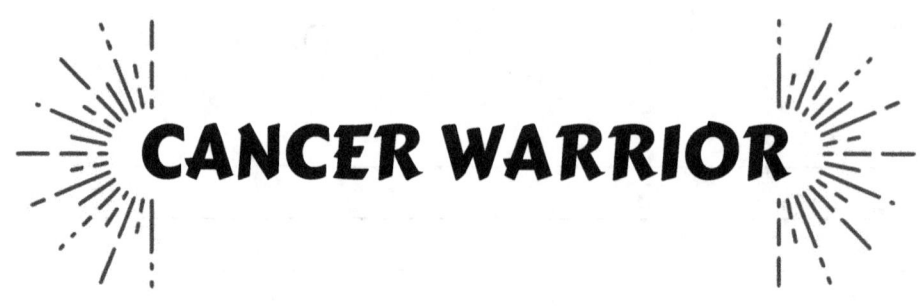

Now that you have dealt with cancer, what three things would you tell a person who just learned of their cancer diagnosis?

Date:_____

Date:_____

_____
_____
_____
_____
_____
_____
_____
_____
_____
_____
_____
_____
_____
_____
_____
_____
_____
_____
_____
_____
_____
_____
_____
_____
_____
_____

**STAY STRONG   BE SAD   SCARED   BE MAD
BE WORRIED   SELF-ACCEPTING   BE POSITIVE
CALM   FIGHT   PATIENT   CONFUSED   ANGRY
DON'T QUIT   BE STRONG   CONTENT   COMMITTED**

Cancer changes you, makes you slow down and re-think things. What are some things you have always wanted to do? Start your life list and do them!

MY LIFE LIST

THINGS I WILL DO THIS YEAR *DONE*

_____ ☐

_____ ☐

_____ ☐

_____ ☐

_____ ☐

_____ ☐

_____ ☐

_____ ☐

_____ ☐

_____ ☐

www.ingramcontent.com/pod-product-compliance
Lightning Source LLC
Chambersburg PA
CBHW062205100526
44589CB00014B/1967